Co-Hearing

Kirk Lumpkin

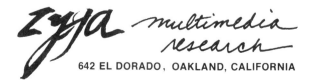

zyga multimedia research

642 EL DORADO, OAKLAND, CALIFORNIA

ACKNOWLEDGEMENTS

Grateful acknowledgement is extended to the editors and publishers of the following publications in which some of these poems have appeared or have been accepted to appear: *City Miner Magazine, Earth First! Newsletter, How Shall The Animal* (anthology), *The Bay Area Poets Coalition's Poetalk-Poemphlet* and *BAPC II* (anthology), *Wayside Poetry Forum, The Margarine Maypole Orangoutang Express,* and *ZYGA Assemblage.*

Library of Congress Cataloging in Publication Data

```
Lumpkin, Kirk, 1951–
   Co-hearing.

   Poems.
   I. Title.
PS3562.U469C6   1983       811'.54          82-61788
ISBN 0-9608438-0-9 (pbk.)
```

Front and back cover photos and
   photo and design for page 37 by Bebe Bertolet

Drawings on pages 12 and 35 Copyright © 1983 by Mary Connolly

Bebe Bertolet, Art Production Consultant

Stephen LaPorta, Copy Editor

Typeset by Eileen Ostrow at the West Coast Print Center,
Berkeley, CA 94703

CONTENTS

Starting Out

Entering Experience

awake!   almost allover
phosphorescent on blue-black snow
self a trembling energy flow
poised, long moments at sea-flank precipice
                feathering air, claws gripped in,,
                                at home

becoming a dark electric waterfall
                    pulse-pouring over the edge
diving in splashing forms of:
                    fingers, hands, arms, legs
                torso, intestines, genitals, hairs
                extending-glass-bead-froth-tips
                dancing branches in starry air
                    over stone-hugging moss

a spirited muscular stretch
                    rooting rushing tendrils
                    in braided cat-
                                a-
                                    racts,
exploding drops in a pool
on the bone-rocks   ringing

later to climb back up
                    seeking sunlight,
re-coiling a cold, dark spring,
and high in treetop perch
    among convoluted clouds
fighting the empty fear of falling,
            of failing, of flying,
        of opening and extending

at last letting go
                to come again
flying through the air's body
a wind of blood and bones
out of the silence   singing

Kirk*

The deep colors of stained glass windows
  in a green meadow
              by a shading grove
Warm flesh and fur that asks
                and gives thanks
                        for food
Bright blood dripped on polished brass spheres
           or on broken bronze spears
The feel of dry rocky dirt
        watered
            by a few tears
The taste of salt, acorns, red wine,
      raw meat, and whole grain
The sound of wood cracking
  or the wind over dry hills
        rattling the leaves of live oak trees,
  or the curling shrieks of circling hawks
The cool smile of the moon
      splashing in the waters of a deep lake
      spreading waves over old, old stone
      on the floor of a cave,
              or a cathedral
      where lions of sunlight are dreaming
      about what they might do
              tomorrow

*kirk means church.

8

Verse/Re-verse Mantra*

Now-Here
Know-Here
Know-Where
You-Are
Some-Where
On-Way
To-Know
All-That
It-Is
In-Here
Out-There
Each-Place
We-Are
Here-Now

*This poem is meant to be read several times in succession: first line through last line, then last line through first line, then first line through last line, then last line through first line, etc.

untitled

in the place   that is my self
i too glow
        with unique madness.
here on the continent's edge
among the dark forms of the sunset city,
in its cooly burning night,
i too
    can stand apart
                    and shine
as do you,
        you star-bodied perverse angels
living in houses
            leaning on other houses
  (few of which you own);
living with the little myths
                and labels
  we enfold each other in
  (warm, sheltered,
                hopefully healing,
                and not too limited)
while a moving history
                is intricately written
in our beautiful scars and wrinkles.

perhaps we find more knowledge
  the farther from sanity we get.
and maybe we must learn more
  than we would ever wish to know.
but some time
            each
                must be left whistling
    (inner flame flickering)   in the awesome stillness,

waiting

for a dark,
        familiar stranger
you think might meet you
                    there

Playin' Jazz

The jazz
          players
          have to get out-
                          Side
                          the sensitive
                                          Wild
                                          music in-
                                                          Side (yeah)
And band
          together
          just to keep sani-
                          Ty
                          in this socie-
                                          Tease
                                          crazed "reali-
                                                          Ty"
OOOh, and   SomeTimes   Got To
smoke-screen-needle-pop-down-golden-mirror-finish-eyelids
meditation   practice   work

                          to keep
                          open
                          to flowing
                          patterns of ex-
                          static
                          sound
Tuning   Being   Being   Tunes
                          outsideinsideout
                          living
                          music

Singing through The changes

Making   real   imaginations   feel

Making   real   imaginations   feel
Feel imaginations   making real
Real   feel-making   imaginations
Imaginations   feel real   making
Making imaginations   real feel
Feel real   making   imaginations
Imaginations making feel   R E A L

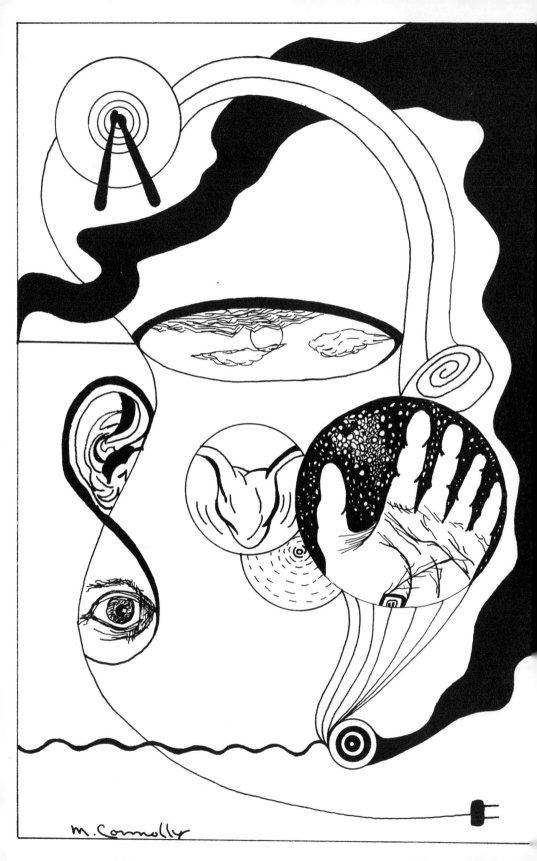

M. Connolly

untitled

is it my art
   that things outside
   find resonance
                    within,
or is it that i
   shape-shake the world
   with my meaning?
do I drum new life into dead skins,
or do i take life
   from the resonant touch
   of skins that once clothed
                    a fellow mammal?

i'm a deranged arranger
                    of organic organization,
a ringer of words
   pounding out a meaning
   in my dull brain;
beating-repeating
   fragments
            of articulation;
trying to clarify,
               energize;
use writing
         to help transform
   inner voice
            into actual sound.

my poems become:
               a singing,
               a purring,
a vibration struck up in the chest,
the measures of the pleasure of the heart.

let my poems live for you.
they can be:
a choir of inner angels,
breaths of mind,
communion with the wind,
food for the spirits of the blood,
indigestible mysteries—jewels you can't remember eating
                    turning up in your turds,
the voices of tiny growing things
                  the human ear
                  can't normally hear,
maps to the places dreams live
               while we're awake,
clouds of new imaginings
   about to rain wisdom,
and promises
   worth keeping.

untitled

Love the Questions
    without attachment to the answers;
you will find enough of what you need.
    so Embrace the Fullness,
    Be your Beliefs.
why not Enjoy
                the Stretching Strain of Mystery?
move in Fantastic Forgiving Faith
    gently Fucking Fickle Fate.

Bust Lust on the Bus
or
Horny on Muni

O the ripple of her nipples
                through her blouse
Want to touch those tender mountains
                at my house

Smitten

she sits in class
   doing nothing
            in particular,
not knowing—
        how
           (exquisitely)
                  she hurts me,
        how
           her loveliness
               wounds me,
        how
           she ravishes
               my imagination.

i want to light up my life
by stealing her beauty
   because i'm afraid
           that stealing
               is the only way
   i could ever hold
           her beauty close.
   because i am shy
           and know she already has
           another man,
i'll try to forget
         (this heart-throb bullshit),
but
   the contours of her face,
   the silken drifts of her hair,
   the fruit firm curves of her breasts,
   the gentle lines of her mouth,
   the quick daisies of her eyes,
   the pastel ring of her voice,
are
   such soft tools
to have cut so deep.

I Want You

out of the blue
   of my life
I don't know what to tell you
   about who
          I am
or how to
       share
   these feelings.

if I could unroll green valleys
   to happily-ever-after in,
would you want me
            then?
(but i can't)

i don't know what i have to offer.
sometimes i feel like:
a short-circuited robot,
or a dead animal by the road,
sometimes a lonely fire in the night,
a trembling prude,
or an utterly voluptuous lover,
a dumb accident,
or a god,
a liberated person,
or a man trapped in himself,
a beat bum,
or a hippie derelict,
or a well-mannered savage,
a world citizen,
or wealthy American,
a renaissance man,
or a master of nothing,
an artist,
or a dilettante,
a meditator on the wisdom of the ages,
or an efficiency expert
   on the best ways
   to waste time,

a cowering paranoid,
or Gaia's brave warrior,
an offbalance juggler of musical spheres,
a new wave tree worshiper,
a believer in all religions,
or a believer in none,
the priest of a faith
                    no one follows,
or a poet
          talking a song
                        of forgotten dreams.

I have imagined myself
   in these roles
   and many others
but I don't know
               who i am,
and I don't know
               who you are.
but that doesn't make me
                      want you
                              any less

Letter From A Shipwrecked Sailor
for P. S.

I.
caught on-in the frantic, hungry
                              unhurried wave
    that hurled me, unfurled me
                        into you.
i sometimes sank
    with flailing fingers
                        or frozen hand upon the rudder,
sometimes sailed the foamy peaks
    feeling the way through
                        with my seaman's blind oar,
now i'm a slightly shaken sailor
                        tossed off your body's shore.

our exposed edges: tattered sails
                              burn with sunset,
riptide through my heart
                        splintering on the rocks.

my love must drift until smoother,
    then leave the lonely grind
                              of salt wet sand,
        climb the cliff,
become a twisted cypress
    standing up again
                        to fight the wind.
but part must also flow-t off in waves
and part root-grasps deep calm—
native at last.

II.
though easier to take our differences
    when i hoped you wanted all of me,
i don't want my jealousy
                            to make us both suffer.
my love for you (i honestly believe)
                has never diminished
    but only changes the mode of its expression.
no reason to let all the tension go slack
                            in the gut-mind-spirit line
    held taut between us.
    but take a few steps back— s t r e t c h —
retaining sufficient tightness
    to play a lively tune upon it,
    to still dance delightfully together
        though in wider circles sailing—
loving
    even without sex
    even if we never see each other.

i thank you for bringing part of me out of hiding.
i hope you learn something from me
though i often failed
    faced with the fiery response-ability
    you laid on me.
i gave-give as best i could-can.

please help me (when and if you can)
    to rise above the facts
that even though you are no longer my lover,
    and are not my mother, a siren,
    the bitch goddess, nor the white goddess
still—
sister, my words
                shipwreck
                        at your feet.

Be My Muse

Please teach me   the language of love.
Let me feel
          how your tongue
                  shapes it.
Teach me the subtle braille
                of your body
   and the sweet lies.
Initiate me in your mysteries—
For I want to enter your life
Like one enters the world
               that a song is—
Not like the listener enters
             (simply engulfed),
But like the musician enters,
  totally intent
         on making the song
               good.

Blessings and Protests

THE PLEDGE OF A HUMAN ANIMAL,
OF A BLOODY SMILING FOOL

I will not be
              a drone of industry
              an oily machine cog
              a devoed clone
              or a plastic mannequin
I will not be a polished steel ball
              in some multinational corporation's
                            giant pinball game
              with nothing
                but electronic bleeps repeating
              in my wired robot brain
I will not let my thoughts be programmed
              by TV consumption jingles
I will not cheerfully join
                            the disco-mechano lockstep
                            toward doom
I will live
              in protest of chemical poisons
                            nuclear weapons and reactors
              until they are stopped
                            or made safe
              or i am split
                            like an atom
Part of me becoming unbelievably beautiful
              part burning unbearably powerful
My mutant cells growing wilder
                            than my own imagination

Marriage Song
*for Rees and Riina**

Brother, we have taken our stumbling dance
                    to cold peaks;
We have greeted warm wave
               on tropic sands;
We have walked dry and lonely worlds together;
We have (w)rung rainbows
                from the clouds of conversations;
We have been embodied angels
   eating dust, smoke, chemicals, and microorganisms;
We have given
         and gathered
                each other's gifts.

Sister, take this man, give this man;
Freshen his dreams;
Help him give birth to a greater Love
   to be his-your own
              without owner;
I am sure lady, you have known pain too,
   bitter darkness
           and bleeding days,
But do not dwell on those,
   dwell in Love's House
            without walls.

Together
Weave a blanket
          from the vineyards' heat-shimmered air
(Wrap it warmly 'round you both);
 Weave a tale
          from the Valley's thick winter fog—

*My friend Rees Nielsen farms grapes for raisins in the San Joaquin Valley near Selma, California, "The Raisin Capitol of the World." Rees and Riina were married October 17, 1977.

24

Wear it as a cape.

Walking lightly
               as you farm the earth
In-jest
     in-earnest
          enjoying
              Her fruits;
Each is a hungry prayer
             that's found rebirth.
Plant the love-seed—
           in the dark night grow bright.
Be green fires reflecting the sun;
Hold your ground against storm, blight, and agribusiness;
Be fountains of joy welling up to the touch
  watering the bodies' needing roots;

And even if the climate turns more arid
  and the Valley dries up
  the wine of life will remain;

And if you age, wrinkling like raisins,
May you laugh at how sweet you've grown.
For there is nothing greater
  through the cycles of the seasons
  the whole earth 'round
Than the Love that turns life sweet.
We have no more
          but work, play,
  and the single spirit
            of our separate
                songs

Swearing

Oh Shit!   Oh God!

and here
           i
              am

somewhere between

but as surely as I've touched the One
I've also touched the Other

though it's nothing to my credit
    when I acknowledge with a curse
it does feel a little better
    when I've turned it into verse

this is my life
    oh god, oh shit
I'll do my best
    to honor it

for Ron McKernan*
March 9, 1973

Pig Pen is dead.
He won't be playin' in the band again.

In the give and take
   there always comes a time for death.
But you get all you need,
All you got to have.

And I'm grateful for the pleasure his singing gave.
His Song lives on tape, on vinyl,
   in the mind,
   and in the rhythms of our bodies
   beyond the grave.

I don't care where he came from,
I don't care where he's goin',
Just as long as he was doin' it right.

And now
       open up and
             Let It Shine
From the Ship of the Sun
             where the grateful dead
             are always making music
For the grateful living
        sitting, standing,
        walking, dancing
               in the sunshine

*Formerly a living member of the Grateful Dead.

we, the churches

in the garden of the world;
we
   are the churches—
the building-bodies
   held
by the unseen hands
          of gravity.

our eye-windows opening,
lungs lofting message,
ribs arching
        above sanctuaries
  where communion food becomes
  pure energy,
hands re-pair in prayer,
our feet: a living foundation.

when hearts pump love
      we voice a true compassion—
the light
      of flame-tongued altar candles.
when (despite our pain) we sing,
    and spread life's celebration,
    the choir master's keyboard
      through our every organ hums
    and blessings start to ring out
      from the belfries of our skulls.

consciousness is a cross: pain + liberation.
we must know
       our lives
         are stained;
by color
    and bars of metal
  from one another
we
  are divided.
yet each is a congregation
         of living cells,
when seen through the spirit's prism—
    a lovely rainbow vision
    not
      a prison.

MONOCULTURE *

MONOLITHIC SKYSCRAPERS,
_____ CONCRETINS_____
OF HOMOGENIZED BOULDERS;
THE LANDSCAPE OF WRECK-TANGLES,
A MONOTONY OF SQUARISM,
THE MONOTONE OF AUTO DRONE
IN DA(I)LY CITY, USA
WHERE NEAT ROWS
OF TICKY-TACKY BOX-HOUSES
BLEND INTO
      THE NAMELESS MARKERS
      OF THE MILITARY CEMETERY.

TV, AN UNSUCCESSFUL OMNIVORE,
SUCKS COLORLESS ENERGY
FOR THE NONSTOP STARE OF ITS
      SEDATIVE RAYGUN,
FOR THE MONOCHROME BUZZ
  OF ITS MONOPOLISTIC LANGUAGE.

ONE ANSWER MEN
SHATTER
      THE ECHOING ORBITS
FOR A SINGLE POWER SOURCE,
TO HOLD A SUN IN THEIR HANDS;
BE WHITE LIGHT BLINDED
IN A UNIVERSE
      THAT CIRCLES AROUND
THEM.

HOLDING INSURANCE POLICIES ON
PLASTIC ASSEMBLY LINE FUTURES
WE'RE DRIVEN ON
THROUGH A GREAT DIVERSITY OF
MAN-YOU-FRACTURED POSSIBILITIES
INTO VAST FIELDS
      OF SAMENESS
BATHED
      IN POISONS,
PRODUCING
      STRONGER INSECTS,
      WEAKER PEOPLE,
      ADDICTED PLANTS.

OUR CULTURE   HAS MONO.

*This term originated in the field of agri-business and refers to single-crop farming.

Tears of White Jade

Jade is the fairest of stones. It is endowed with 5 virtues: charity is typified by its lustre, bright yet warm, rectitude by its translucency revealing the color and markings within, wisdom by the purity and penetrating quality of its note when this stone is struck, courage in that it may be broken but can not be bent, equity in that it has sharp angles which injure none. — Confucious

My tears are white jade,
Frozen inside my eyeballs
Before they can ever come out.
And though they be warm and glistening
They *are* hard tough rocks
       all the same.
I have been taught that it is right for a man
  in this culture,
Even when alone,
To clench his sorrow, his emotions, his loving gentleness
  this way.

Is there no way for an American male to really let flow
  and mingle his with the lives of others?

Yes, for there are times when even rock melts,
As there are times when mountains burst up in one's path,
And a volcano overflows redness like a stabbed artery
Sending a river of lava to cool in the ocean's salty waves;
The Earth's own anguished laughter shaking-quaking the land,
  cracking pipes and dams,
         rechanneling water;
Or as in the warming spring sun—
  even thorny cacti flower
       and drip with nectar;
So in time
    a too-little used cup
       tightly held,
         within atremble,
  too full,
    too long,
      runneth over.
And hot liquid frees itself
From being locked
    in white rocks.

War Is A Wonderful Thing

War is a wonderful thing
because it's like a syringe
   in the bloodstream
                of the economy
because it makes boys
            into robot-men

War is a wonderful thing
because it affords a chance
               for the most foolish forms
   of heroism
        to be exhibited
because it proves which nation can most quickly become
   insensitive toward the people of another nation

War is a wonderful thing
because it inspires scientists
   to create technological marvels
   like napalm and nuclear weapons
because it gives the freedom to lawfully murder

War is a wonderful thing
because the vague softness of kindness
   is eclipsed by the focussed hardness of hate
because it's something we can all rally around,
   really get together on

War is a wonderful thing

The Seven Lakes of Band-I-Amir

I.
The azure lakes of Band-I-Amir
   are a bracelet of lapis lazuli
   gleaming in the sun,
Flung there in the canyon dust
   by some joyous goddess—
A gift left in her dervish dance
For the nomads
          in the arid
             Afgan
               highland.

II.
Just down the valley
          (in a later age)
Monks honeycombed the cliffs
   with cells and sanctuaries,
Carved colossal statues of the Buddha,*
   painted murals,
   and tended the jeweled garden
             of the Void.

But the peace of this place is shattered again:
Where Genghis Khan came slaughtering,
And conquering emperor Aurangzeeb
   smashed the statue faces;
Now Russian imperialists
            stalk the land,
The Moslem villagers must meet fear
   and fight
       for what is theirs,
The caves are empty (or hiding places),
And the faceless giants
          still look
          to the distant jagged peaks
          of the Hindu Kush.

*The tallest statues of Buddha in the world—one 175-ft. and another 120-ft. tall.

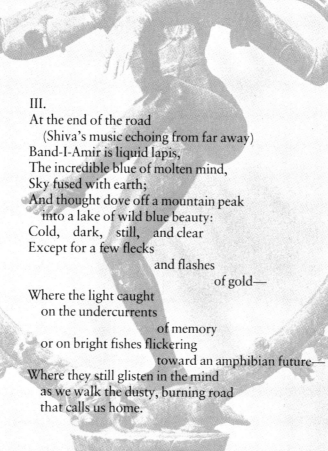

III.
At the end of the road
   (Shiva's music echoing from far away)
Band-I-Amir is liquid lapis,
The incredible blue of molten mind,
Sky fused with earth;
And thought dove off a mountain peak
   into a lake of wild blue beauty:
Cold,   dark,   still,   and clear
Except for a few flecks
                        and flashes
                                    of gold—
Where the light caught
   on the undercurrents
                        of memory
   or on bright fishes flickering
                        toward an amphibian future—
Where they still glisten in the mind
   as we walk the dusty, burning road
   that calls us home.

Go from Regret to the Magic Worlds

when the heart holds grief too close
let pain become an axis
drawing 'round it
the scabd burnd scard darkness

turn it deep   turn it round
till it cuts open a space
where the magic worlds can grow
        and spin out of us   again

        the magic worlds
that are (hidden)
        in each moment,
        in every thing

and some things
                like the flowers
can no longer stand
        to hold these worlds within
and they run across their petal-faces
in foolish pollen-planet grins

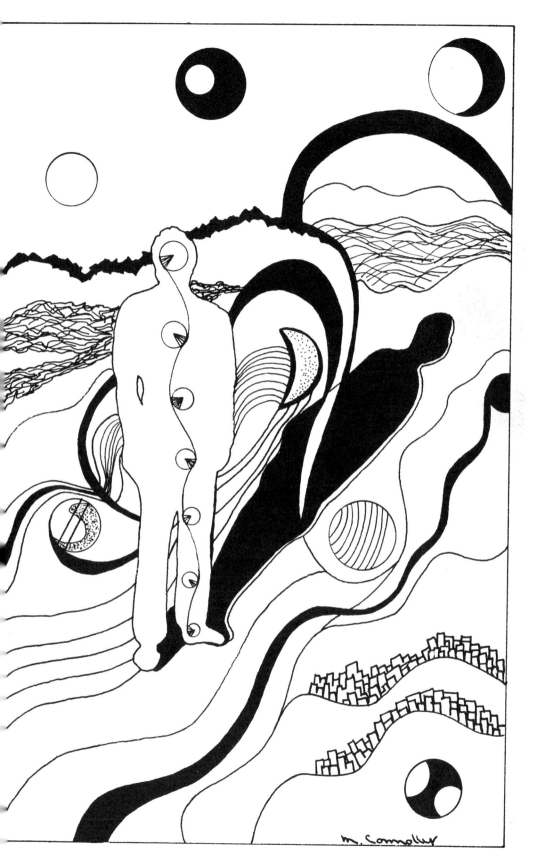

Dancing Fills Us
With Exquisite Emptiness

the party may seem
                          almost over
      but it has just condensed
booze and food almost gone
      the fleshy and liquid bittersweet
      eaten, drunken up
full but light
                          a dedicated few
                                          dance on
hearts beating liquid rhythms
climbing the winding fountain of the blood
            blown by the wind of each other's
      swirling dance
accented by the clap of flesh
                                          backed by bones
            sweet heels tatooing the floor
workin' it up
                          playin' it down
their erratic butterfly flight
                  on the turbulent wings of
      champagne, cocaine, coffee, and grass
                  may make them appear
                                          like the lunatic fringe
      but these people
                          form the hard-core
                          getting smoother
wreck-less bodies
                          (of bending boughs
      and juicy redness)
                          whirling around
            the center   they seek
(without thinking   that they seek it)
      organs orbiting   the hollow hub
      that fills them   with a vibrant hum
      of soundless   singing
      for it is from this   opening center that
)though   empty(
            the song   comes
born of the supple joining
                  of opposing tensions
this dark meat-cave
            of birth and death
      is filled with moving lights
      made by rubbing our magic lamps together
      calling up love's body laughter
Oh this   swinging   ringing   bell of   being

untitled

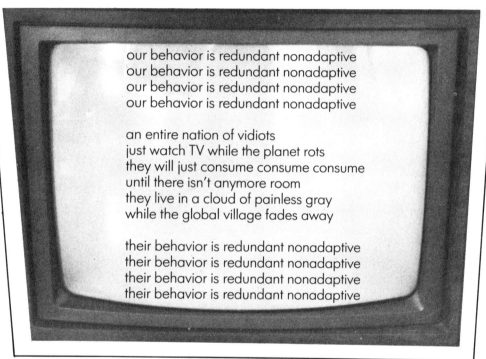

our behavior is redundant nonadaptive
our behavior is redundant nonadaptive
our behavior is redundant nonadaptive
our behavior is redundant nonadaptive

an entire nation of vidiots
just watch TV while the planet rots
they will just consume consume consume
until there isn't anymore room
they live in a cloud of painless gray
while the global village fades away

their behavior is redundant nonadaptive
their behavior is redundant nonadaptive
their behavior is redundant nonadaptive
their behavior is redundant nonadaptive

turn off the TV
and (tell   a   vision)

of your own

The Voice

Listen
for there is a Voice
from the wilderness outside
                    and inside;
a Voice
        that no one owns.

And we have an emptiness
    far deeper than wanting,
where quavering with need
    the tongueless blood can't cry out for love,
where caged animals pace,
where possible saints gag on self-pity,
where sugar-coated angel tongues
    have lost the power to sing,
where icy societal mirrors
    make our own bodies ugly,
where rain aches
    in dehydrated clouds,
where ears filled with static ego signals
    are turning into pavement,
where stone wisemen
    grit their teeth,
where freedom wants to dance
                            and ring its bells
    but shakes only
            with fear.

Listen,

Peace,

Be
Still
for you will not be
                        (full-filled)
until
the Voice
at the heart of silence

                    (   )

is heard

Gila Songs

An Interlude

simply marvelous

frog egg strands
caught on
     submerged branches
          and rocks,
trans-parent tube-sacks
filled with black seeds
undulating
     in the river's
clear
    current

untitled

Gila Wilderness, New Mexico

walking up/down mountains--
pine needle soft
                    and rock-hard paths.
slogging with booted feet
    through clear-cold streams
    in the eroded depths of canyons.
while in these wilds
    we are a new
    but temporary tribe.
we carry our culture
    packed on our backs,
    packed in our minds.
mostly
        we think in words,
        walk inside ideas.
when we sleep
                    we put down a foam pad
                    between us
                                and the earth,
                    we dream in warmth
                    wrapped in synthetic cloth.
still
    we take on the challenges,
    begin to take in the lessons
    of the stone cliffs we climb;
    sometimes nakedly touching nature
        and each other.
beaten on the hard hills
    till (in a faltering
                    human way)
    we are able to meet the measure
    of a stronger, tougher,
    longer-lasting
                    music

ALL: the heart's song

all that can move
                          love to dance
all that have voice
                          love to sing
all that can hear
                          love to listen
all that can see
                          love the light
all that know joy
                          love to live
all that have life
                          love to love

The Last Night and Morning
for K.H.

Southwest Outward Bound School
Gila Wilderness, New Mexico

evergreen clearing   bright moon,
            you
           even more lovely
           silvered
          with this light.

you bless me
          with the touch
   of your long lean smooth strong body.
we make love
          (almost as gracefully
             as our connected bags allow).
deliciously sizzling in your gentle fire
my ideas of love dissolve
   and slowly trickle a-way
   into dark woods

   growing under silent peaks.

everyone else seems asleep.

a whippoorwill sounds in the stillness.

we smile
and also claim a place in the night
with our sweet (but quieter) song.

i trembling whisper my desire
not to have you
           walk out of my life tomorrow.

gazing at stars and eyes
we talk, savor,
   caress, and
   hold our warmth of loving,
                  till
   reluctantly
we curl into sleep

and rise in the pre-dawn darkness
    only when the bottom of our bag is shaken
    interrupting our last bare hugs.
we shiver into clothes,
separate our bags,
quickly finish packing,
go to the dirt road to run 10 miles.
i want to win this race
for me—
            but also for you
perhaps because in some (absurdly macho) way
i want to prove i'm good enough for you.
and thoughts of you give me strength;
inside as i run i name you: my Lady of the Pines
    (last night haloed with seed-bearing cones)
                name you: Lady Long Legs
    (picturing shapely calves
                            on wilderness paths).
love is an engine in my heart—
sun rising,
        my body striding
inside a happy Gila monster
    fiercely bites its own tail,
    becomes a flaming wheel—ball lightning,
    breath a softly rolling thunder.
i've never run so well before—fast and pleasurable.
only the instructors are faster.

then a bus ride and last goodbyes
                            before your flight.

now, a whole continent
            and more   stretches   between us,
but for a few moments
on this little page (this stage)
i become the poem,
make love to you
            with words.

Spirals

a spiral fire links these lines
to blood-roots running deep,
though fear and pain oppress at times
the Vision never sleeps

The Wild Creatures of My Childhood*

I. Perhaps of all the wild creatures
                    native to my childhood
        it is the vulture
        that now sways most powerfully
        in the unseen wilderness
                        of my imagination.
        But I do not know, I cannot know.
                    I speak in darkness
                    hoping that for an instant
                    the words will illuminate
                    some of the shadowy forms.
        So many times I saw those dark lords
            wheeling majestically in the sky
            shadowing the ground.

        Then the hawk appealed to me more:
            smaller, more handsome,
            a sleek diver of contained storm fury,
            a predator, not a scavenger,
            and seen more rarely.
        There were prettier birds
            with lovelier songs,
            but they usually seemed puny
            compared with hawk and buzzard
            (not the material for a powerful totem).
        Me and the other boys used to yip and howl
            like we thought coyotes did,
            but we never saw 'em.
        I liked to watch lizards basking in the sun,
            liked to try to catch them;
            caught a lot
                    but missed most.
        (The blue-bellied ones were the best to look at.)
        I would hold them in my hands a short time
            then let them go.

*I lived most of the first 12 years of my life in San Benancio Canyon between Monterey and Salinas, California. Behind our house was "The Hill" where I was first alone with Nature.

Horny toads were fascinating to look at
    but after awhile were really too easy to catch.
Rarer to catch and see were snakes;
    (that strange phallic power
     coiled
            within me).
One time holding a small gopher snake,
    I let my grip relax on its wriggling strength,
    it bit me right between the eyebrows,
    which hardly hurt
                        but drew blood.
Once I caught a king snake,
    thought its black/white splotches beautiful.
Not till years later did I see a rattler in the wild;
    but there was always a scary thrill
    in just thinking about catching snakes;
    I gazed long at their pictures in books.
I caught tadpoles
    and watched them magically transform into frogs
    (when they lasted that long).
I had pet newts, named Eggy and Gramps,
    but no one wanted to pet them;
    they just sat in the aquarium
                        bored
    or eating their ration of ant eggs.
There was the soft whirrrrr
    of quail coveys in flight.
    I caught a baby quail once, brought it home,
    but my mother made me take it back.
    I thought it died but hoped better.
    (That was in the field
     where they grew strawberries,
     where there are condos now.)
Gophers were seldom seen
    and when they were they were usually dead.
There were only a few places nearby
    where deer were often seen;
    more often their tracks and scats.
Sometimes I would see them out the school bus window
    running through sunlight and live oak shade
    on the Marcus Ranch.

Mountain lions were only a glorious day dream.
  I would love to have come 'round a bend
  and been face to face
  with that locus of savage power;
  a thing made of sunblasting granite,
  its roar the only wind.

Perhaps the fascination I feel for vultures
  comes from seeing them so often,
  but never up close, never to touch;
  the everpresent feeling their distance gave
  and not a death wish
                that intrigues me now.
These living gliding compost heaps
  still soar high, wild, and free—
                    dark against the sky,
Recycling through their tearing beaks
  turning the dead into fresh clean flesh.
Maybe they'll be the last animals to go.
Maybe they're the heralds of a new species.
For there is surely something
                in that patient circling.

II. *envoy*
  old buzzard, old turkey vulture of my spirit
    eat up that which dwelling on pain brings
    eat up the dross
    eat up the dead
    eat up the useless
    eat up the wasteful
    eat up the cancer
    eat up the anti-life
    eat it up mercilessly
  Oh scavenger of joy
    discover the food the too proud would leave behind
    that we may grow strong
    circling again
        flying higher

RECYCLE

we grow
                   between rot and rebirth;
fertilized by all we experience.
this earth (the house we live in)
can be a place of beauty
and we are worse off
                              when we turn it into trash.
so in service
              of the slow work
                              of the natural cycles
do the Dance that makes us whole;
recycling the ugliness, the useless;
take it personally:
Recycle your trash
Recycle your glass
Recycle your cans
Recycle your news
Recycle your shit
Recycle your thoughts
Recycle your flesh
Recycle your blood
Recycle your hate
Recycle your love
RECYCLE NOW!

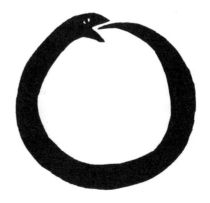

winter solstice-christ mass poem

the sun labors into the year's longest darkness;
it sinks in red now,
                          to rise toward spring.
traveling into late hours,
when few if any other people
                                still seek home or haven
in the cold desert night,
a couple finally finds shelter;
kind people let them rest
                          among their gentle beasts.
in this protective warmth
                                the pregnant woman gives birth,
bears up in the opening deliverance;
a baby of flesh and spirit emerges
and the world shines anew
                          in its eyes.

a light snow covers everything;
the morning sun is magnified in a mirror of crystals;
the white winter rose has bloomed.
standing as silent guardian
                                over the ground,
on which new groves will sprout
                                where the old rotted,
is the forevergreen tree, born of sky and earth,
                                the Tree of Life.
from it the creative carpenter carves with care,
a place for love to flourish,
in the trunk of that living thing
                                that keeps on growing
despite the world's
                          knives and nails.

Vernal Equinox
3:10 am, March 20, 1980

In minutes we will be exactly halfway
On our yearly trip
                    from the darkest night
                        to the lightest day.
Hesitation---pacing---   arguing with myself:
            to go outside or not?

I go for it, out the door, to the Panhandle's end.
            Hesitate again---is farther worth the effort?
            ---cars go by---
            a jogger across the street (!)--
            sea-born breeze in my face—

Head on into The Park
                    (Coltrane's tune "Equinox"
                    blowing inside me
                    booodahdaaaah boodahdaaaaah . . . . .)
Turn up side path
                    (wind hush waft of thick flower perfume
)Step softly
            under overhanging boughs
            fantasizing wino violence
            or a raccoon/startled as me.
Breathe deep—   sigh   hummmmmm—
Out of sight of lights
                    turn eyes to stars.
Look up through big-limbed sycamore tree
            its beauty
            of irregular
            sky-earth grasping
                            symmetry—
And dizzy with upward looking,
                            get dizzier still
    with a whirling armspread dervish dance.
Then back toward street lights;
    the crash of garbage trucks.
Just ahead a cop rolls down Hayes St.
                            U turns/stops
                            waits/for me (?)

I hope not.
It's no crime to walk late in The Park.
But I tremble a little;
Getting to the cop --
                    he's out, making notes.
He looks up, I smile, he nodssays "Hi."
I say "Hi. Happy Spring --
                    Spring officially started at 3:10."
He says "Really?"
I walk on smiling.

But for a few moments
                    I feared his power;
Like my fear in the dark park,
Only different.
We fear each Other, we fear the Law, we fear Nature.
Our personal powers go unrecognized
                              or misused.
But I hope with this Spring (as I guess I always hope)
That my life will be better,
That we will grow deeper in the Laws of Love and Nature.
And though it may be a fool's hope
I love its expectant giddy balance,
Love the dance of Day and Night,
Love the seasons' cycles,
Love the crazy human scene,
Love to voice the vision,
Love to sing
            the green blood's song

Co-Hereing

co-hearing
in a body of silence:
   One clear stream
               Centered everywhere
   vibrating with all the ecoing systems
   (plants-animals-computers-constellations-cities-watersheds-
reading
the body of being:
   the real book of Here,
   the information in a living bristlecone pine,
   in the contours of a hill or a lover,
   in the patterns of flowers or streets
writing-speaking-singing
a body of sound-words:
   tiny energy catalysts
   forming noise into new meaning,
   sparkling naked wit,
   communicating love

nourished by the richness of the diverse community,
   which is the total energy field,
together let us ride
   the widening gyres
               of positive feedback loops
into a cultural climax forest—
   into a subtly electric
               wilderness

where tools-toys—our technology
   meets the natural place
using the civilized and wild
   we'll work-play on the interface

engaging in:
   SYMBIOTIC SYNERGETIC BIOFEEDBACK CYBERNETICS
   SYMBIOTIC SYNERGETIC BIOFEEDBACK CYBERNETICS

and
   Listening
to our relatives in Life:
   Man Kind, Woman Kind, People Kind, Mammal Kind,
   Bird Kind, Reptile Kind, Amphibian Kind,
   Anthropod Kind, Mollusc Kind, Fish Kind,
   Insect Kind, Bacteria Kind, Plant Kind
   All That Is
   Being Kind
for each has a song:
                arriba-deva-bebop
                  like-me-and-you
                a-blue-rockin'-pain-stop
                  a-jingling-goo

Be You
Be you
it is Be-You-tiful
Be-You-ti-Full
Beauty-Full
Oh so Beautiful
O—O—O—
        O
     TO   BE
     TO   BE
     AS   IS
      A
      S

      I
      S
BREATHING-GROWING
     AIR THAT SINGS
            GROOOWING GROOOOOWING
            Growing into
                Every thing

Condensing Exaltation Mantra

Exalt your Being in the Immensity of Isness
Exalt your Being in Immensity of Isness
Exalt Being in Immensity of Isness
Exalt Being Immensity of Isness
Exalt Being Immensity Isness
Exalt Being Isness
Exalt Being
Exalt

Contorted Light

All life on this planet is made from sunlight
which holds the whole food chain together.

I.
after night thundershowers
the dazzle of desert morning
       softly crawls across my eyelids.
i rise stiffly
      to the simple pleasure
             of movement,
squint-smile at the reflection
      of blue sky
          and white moving clouds
      in a mud puddle
      on whose edge a motley spectrum spreads
         on a tiny oil slick.
my brain bubbles in its bone chalice,
my eyes a sparkling libation,
         a toast to the new day.

in a still moment
the soft implosions of dreams
echo again,
      ripple from concentricities
      deep inside—
attentive tissues dance motionlessly
until
   the iridescent hum of a song
           blossom-flows
   through my lips
and i playfully splash the puddle with my hand,
light jumping off in contorted merriment.

this little puddle   that may be burned dry
before moon, stars,   and trembling darkness
once more caress
      this stretch of earth.

II.
the pattern of evolution, on this planet,
    seems to have required:
fire and glaciers,
plants to eat sunlight and exhale air,
plankton floating in oceans
eaten by the giants we call whales,
the countless (unseen) bacteria,
the busy ants and bees,
gentle green vines in loamy soil,
roses and redwoods,
oysters and pearls,
the songs of frogs, doves, and coyotes,
dinosaurs rumbling the earth,
rodents and primates,
snakes curled in dry leaves beneath trees
    or spread on warm rocks in the sun,
antelopes with soft eyes and graceful speed,
dolphins and porpoises,
furry beasts with blood dripping from their teeth,
and the whirling many-sided human mind.

feather-fur-flower-bark-quill-scale-tendril-tentacle-claw-horn
still spiral-dance within us,
yet when a species dies
    even if we never touched them (bodily or mentally)
    we lose a lovely whole.
    a complete way of being
                                vanishes,
    the information they embodied
                                is gone.
for mind and meat
                    wilderness is freedom
and it is not some economic engine, church, or government
    that keeps us going—
    it is Life,
            it is the animals of the blood,
it is their-our diversity
    that feeds thought and physicality.
they-we hold within our every cell
                                the shimmering plasm
    of the rainbow web.

III.
the present devolution
                        is merely one convolution
in the brain of the Life-beast
                        becoming conscious
Our actual future
                is an unimaginable adventure

so for now
            look around

this is the business of why we're here:
to attend to the everyday
                        work-play,
to bend sunlight into new shapes,
to spiral thoughts out into space,
to make tools, use tools and be tools
to dance, sing, sow and build,
to be stewards of the Earth,
to bear the pain
                        creating joy,
to mingle our parents genes with our lovers,
finding pleasure in this pooling
                        from which children spring
   perhaps to mutate
                        toward monster
                                    or toward angel,
to bend slowly into death's caresses
or to have our hearts burst-flower
   in a final terrible ecstacy,
                the CR(I I I I I)Y
                of the Spirit's SOOOOOONG

Note On The Author:

Kirk Lumpkin was born February 4, 1951 in Yuma, Arizona. He lived most of his first 12 years in San Benancio Canyon between Monterey and Salinas, California before moving with his parents to Muncie, Indiana. He returned to California in 1969 to attend the University of the Pacific, under whose auspices he went to study in India in 1970.

Arriving back in the U.S. near the end of the Vietnam War, Lumpkin filed for and received conscientious objector status. To fulfill his alternate service, he went to work at Intersection ("San Francisco's quintessential art center."—*Berkeley Monthly*), where he eventually became theater manager. Here he met saxophonist Dennis Mackler, who collaborated with him on poetry-music pieces. Mackler, Lumpkin, and guitarist Paul Mills have gone on to form the band, DETOUR, in which Lumpkin plays drums and contributes lyrics and vocals.

In 1981, Lumpkin teamed with artist Bebe Bertolet and poet Barbara Gravelle on *ZYGA Assemblage*, a multimedia arts publication about which the press has said:

> " . . . innovative . . . a must for those intrigued by vanguard culture."—*Focus*
> " . . . no description will do it justice. . . . The art of assemblage, of mixed media cross-genre publication achieves a kind of ultimate . . ."—*The Small Press Review*
> " . . . fertile concept"—*Contra Costa Times*
> " . . . outstanding transformation of the magazine format . . . energetic challenge to a stuffy art world."—*Afterimage*

ZYGA Assemblage was on the Selection List of The Small Press Book Club, and a copy of it is in the Bay Area Music Archives.

The author holds a B.A. in Creative and Language Arts from Antioch University/West in San Francisco and a Certificate in Arts Administration and Management from the University of California at Berkeley Extension.

Kirk Lumpkin's poetry broadsides have been exhibited in the Internationalist Arts Festival (Anti-World War 3 and for the Future) and at the Thurman Casey Library, Walnut Creek, California. His broadsides, taped works, *ZYGA Assemblage*, and this book are available from the publisher through which he can also be contacted for readings and workshops.

published by
Zyga Multimedia Research
642 El Dorado Avenue
Oakland, Ca 94611